How to Reach and Achieve a Lifetime of Physical Fitness

By

Okongor Ayuk Ndifon

Usage

You may use this ebook without giving it out and without selling it.

DISCLAIMER AND/OR LEGAL NOTICES:

The information presented herein represents author's view as of the date of publication. Due to the fact that the rate with which conditions change, with the use of the internet, the author reserves the right to alter and update his opinion based on the new conditions. It is hoped that the knowledge gained from this ebook would go along way to helping you adapt to the changing condition of the internet.

The ebook is for information purposes only. While every attempt has been made to verify the information provided in this ebook, the author assume any responsibility for errors, wrong interpretation, or omissions. Any slights of people or organizations are unintentional.

The purchaser or reader of this information is responsible for the use of this material, and there is no guarantee of success in usage. See your family medical doctor or personnel and any other specialist as regards this ebook, for expert advice.]

Contents

Introduction

This book is meant to describe physical fitness, and ways of reaching and achieving a lifetime of physical fitness. You will learn about exercise and its benefits, and how to make exercise a regular habit.

Physical fitness is the ability of one's body to get along with its environment and being able to cope with daily activities.

Physical fitness and good health has been known to emanate from regular and adequate exercise, proper nutrition, reduced or stress free life (adequate rest), cleanliness, proper medication, suitable environment, and a positive mental attitude.

In all the various ways to reaching and achieving a lifetime of physical fitness, having good exercise habits and correct nutrition are keys to physical fitness.

For example, it is known that a regular exercise of 20 to 30 minutes daily for about 5 days in a week is adequate for one to be physically fit.

Regular physical activity is known to decrease high blood pressure, type two diabetes, colon and breast cancer, heart disease, etc.

You can enhance your physical fitness through exercise and thereby become or maintain a healthier life.

For one to be socially, physically, mentally, emotionally, occupationally, and spiritually well, such must be physically fit, avoid risks factors for disease, and show no sign of disease and sickness.

1. Definition and Meaning of Physical Fitness

Physical fitness definition here is very much targeted towards functional ability. We see it as the ability to meet physical challenges, whether related to work, sport, recreation, combat, or other life activities.

A man's physical fitness must be seen in the context of the specific physical challenges he is likely to face. Thus the criteria for a physically fit fire fighter or combat soldier are by necessity much more stringent than those for an elderly, frail man whose daily activities such as climbing stairs, or even getting up out of a chair, are challenging.

There are several components of physical fitness including some that are not readily improved by training, such as coordination, reaction time, peripheral vision, and height.

Since little or nothing can be done to improve these, our physical fitness definition below includes only physical capabilities that are amendable to training. These are strength, muscular endurance, aerobic endurance, speed, agility/quickness, flexibility, and balance:

Physical fitness is one of the important ways of measuring the physical health of an individual. Physical fitness informs us how healthy a person is. Physical fitness affects a person's mental capacity, productivity at work, and stress management.

Physical fitness is a necessity for the mere fact that a person feels better and looks better when they are physically fit.

Physical fitness is commonly defined as the capacity to carry out the day's activities, pursue recreational activities, and have the physical capability to handle emergency situations.

2. Basics of Physical Fitness

There is need to know how you can enter into physical fitness through an understanding of the concept.

Many misconceptions abound concerning the meaning and definition of physical fitness. It is seen by some people to mean being lean or thin and others view fitness as building up one's muscles.

It the actual meaning, physical fitness is being physically fit, normal and suitable. If you are physically fit, you are able to function optimally. It tells how much one is healthy.

Physical fitness is majorly defined as the state or condition of being physically healthy, as a result of exercise, correct nutrition, and enough rest. It is therefore being in a good condition of general well-being, seen in physical soundness and mental balance.

The capacity of the heart, lungs, muscles, and blood vessels, to function optimally, indicates that one is physically fit.

Physical fitness affects one's productivity, mental capacity, immunity, stress management, physical outlook, and a happy state of mind.

When one is physically fit, such is free from illness and able to cope with daily activities without getting tired, enjoys leisure and copes with emergencies.

Components of Physical Fitness

In defining physical fitness, there are varying definitions, largely due to misconception of the term, but it is agreed that there are five basic components of physical fitness, for moderately tasking occupation or lifestyle of an average person.

The basic health related components of physical fitness are body composition, flexibility, muscular endurance, muscular strength, and cardio-respiratory endurance.

The health related components are the major components of physical fitness. Skill related components of physical fitness include balance, power, agility, coordination, speed and reaction time.

Becoming Physically Fit

You can begin to make changes in your life by engaging in physical activity. Most physical exercises can meet the needs of the various components of physical fitness mentioned above.

Get busy on a daily basis with such exercises as recreational swimming, bicycling, jogging, brisk walking, running and your fitness is sure.

Basic Components of Physical Fitness

Complete physical fitness is composed of many components. But for moderately tasking occupation or lifestyle, health related components will do.

Physical fitness is the ability to function and perform effectively in all activities and still have ability to take care of emergencies. There are basically five components of physical fitness as stated below:

Body Composition

This is the ratio of body fat to lean mass (muscle, bone, important tissues and organs). It is not the general body weight.

Flexibility

 This refers to the ability to move joints and stretch muscles through their full range of motion. A flexible individual can easily bend backwards to touch the floor, and can also easily bend forward to touch the toes or floor. Regular stretching increases the range of motion and enables the stimulation of muscle growth.

It is necessary that you stretch your muscles before sleeping, to avoid body pains after waking up. Flexibility helps to prevent injuries.

Muscular Endurance

Muscular endurance is simply the amount of time that one's muscles are able to perform a certain activity before they become tired. It is the ability to repeat a movement many times or to hold some weight at a particular position for a sustained period of time.

Lifting a measured weight for about two minutes or the ability to lift the same weight five or more times is a measure of muscular endurance.

Muscle Strength

Muscle strength is the ability to exert maximum force for a brief time. It is the ability to do some work of maximum intensity at once, such as lifting a heavy object.

Cardio-respiratory Endurance

Other names for this component of physical fitness are aerobic endurance, oxidative endurance, cardio-vascular endurance, or stamina endurance.

Cardio-respiratory endurance is the ability of the lungs and heart to supply sufficient oxygen and nutrients to all parts of the body during physical activity.

It shows how well the heart and lungs work together in carrying out the above task.

The above basic or major components of fitness are health related. Skill related components of physical fitness include balance, power, agility, coordination, speed and reaction time.

Physical fitness is one major way of determining the physical health of an individual. For you to be physically fit, you must pay attention to exercise or regular workouts, correct nutrition, and enough rest.

A fitness program can help maintain all the components of physical fitness through physical training.

You must do away with unhealthy eating habits and avoid sedentary lifestyle.

Types of exercise to help you become physically fit include recreational swimming, jogging, running, stretching, bicycling, and weight lifting.

Benefits of Physical Fitness

We shall now look at the various benefits of physical fitness, indicating how to reap from them.

Physical fitness is the capacity of the muscles, blood vessels, lungs and heart, to function at optimal level. Physical fitness is generally gotten through exercise, proper nutrition, and adequate rest.

As a beginner, start with 15 minutes daily exercise and move up to 30 minutes of daily exercise or physical activity, for at least 5 days a week. Exercises to get started include brisk walking, jogging, stretching, swimming, and bicycling, to help build your physical fitness.

The various benefits of physical fitness include:

Building a Healthy Mind and Good Mental Health

Physical fitness and exercise brings about happiness, a healthy mind, and sound mental health. A healthy mind helps in boosting your inner confidence. Mental health will mean a better performance in academics.

Prevents Disease Attacks

A fitness program will help in building up the immune system. When the immune system is strengthened, it helps in fighting infections and diseases.

Never abandon your health to pursue wealth, because health will surely bring you back.

Good Look and Beautiful Skin

A physically fit body, whose toxins have been detoxified, becomes toned up. This will beautify your skin and give you a good look.

Enhances Your Body Function

The way your heart and lungs function is enhanced through physical fitness.

Exercise and physical fitness improves the flow of blood to the heart through increased intake of oxygen.

Enhances Better Sleep at Night

A good restful sleep a night is made possible through exercise and physical fitness. The quality of your sleep will improve due to increased intake of oxygen, which is why natural deep breathing exercise is very helpful in this regard.

Builds a Healthier Body

Exercise and physical fitness helps one to stay healthy. Physical activity can help you live longer. It can give your body a healthy weight and prevent some diseases.

Physical fitness strengthens your immune system, which in turn fights infections and diseases that can become problems.

 Risks of developing high blood pressure, high cholesterol, diabetes, and cancer, can be reduced through exercise and physical fitness.

There are many more benefits of physical fitness and may include increased flexibility, overall muscle strength, a regulated appetite, stronger bones, improved circulatory system, renewed energy, stress relieve, and fat loss.

Factors Affecting Physical Fitness

There are some major factors affecting physical fitness. These factors need be considered to enable you know how to carry out your physical fitness goals.

Physical fitness vary from one person to another, therefore the following factors that affect physical fitness are:

Present Age

The older the age the lesser the fitness and performance level of an individual. This is because of the degenerative nature of the body at old age.

As one advance in age, the muscles, ligaments and tendons become shorter, joints become worn out, the heart muscles become weak, and bones become brittle.

When physical activity in embraced at early age, it helps to restrict and return these body problems to normal.

Other factors include Hereditary, Diet, Environment, Sex, Physical maturity, Stress, Health problems, and regularity, etc.

3. Ways of Achieving Physical Fitness

There are various ways in which you can achieve Physical Fitness. These include Adequate Exercise, Correct Diet or Nutrition, Enough Rest (Avoid if possible or manage your stress level well), **Cleanliness, Medication, and a Positive Mental Attitude** (Avoid worry and anxiety.).

A. Correct Nutrition and Physical Fitness

A balanced diet is very important in bringing about the wellness and fitness of an individual. To reach and achieve physical fitness, it is therefore important that proper or correct nutrition is adapted on a daily basis.

Exercise alone cannot give physical fitness; proper nutrition must be taken into consideration.

Exercise and Proper Nutrition

Good diet or nutrition and exercise go along together for the good of our bodies. Exercise is going to give us fitness along with four major things: flexibility, strength, muscle endurance, and cardiovascular health.

One thing to remember is that a bad diet can affect the way that your fitness training goes even if you follow the best type of exercise plan that you can.

You need to put a healthy diet and a lot of exercise together to stay as healthy as you can.

How long do you need to exercise to keep as healthy as you can? The average is at least 20 minutes of exercise at least three times a week. This will help to strengthen the cardiovascular health.

Another idea is that 3500 calories must be used in a week by doing any sort of physical activity. This will benefit you and your heart as well. It is good to seek the advice of your doctor first to find out what exercise plan is going to be best for you and your body.

The energy nutrients that are stored like glucose and fatty acids with a few amino acids are let out into the blood during exercise in order to provide energy for what you are doing. This means that the body will respond to exercise by adjusting its fuel amounts.

Experts have made a way to use diet to control high blood pressure and now they are finding out that exercise has a role in keeping blood pressure from increasing.

With the reduction of sodium into your body, weight loss and limited alcohol use, along with the increased amount of physical activity and a low fat diet, you can control hypertension.

To build muscle in the body, proteins are used and this is true when the body is at rest after exercise or any type of physical activity.

For the athletes, the protein amounts are going to be higher. It should be considered that athletes also need more carbohydrates as well. If they do not take in enough carbs, their protein will be used all up for fuel and there will not be anything left for muscle building after exercise is done.

Researches say that weight bearing exercises like walking, dancing, running, sports and so much more, are very good at getting good bone health. Exercise alone cannot make your body healthy.

You need to have the proper calcium and other vitamins and minerals required for bones must go with the adequate amount of exercise to provide the best bone health.

Along with exercise, diet can help keep your body working good and in the right mode for the rest of your life.

Correct Nutrition and a physically fit Heart

Good food for a healthy heart depends on what you eat. Agents responsible for blood vessel damage, cause heart disease. Oxygen in a place where it is not supposed to be found can cause a tendency for it to react with fatty substances and turn them into harmful compounds.

These fats can cause clogging of arteries. Oxidized fats get into the body through two means, in diets or when oxygen reacts with fats in your body.

It is important to cut down on dietary fats, to be able to limit your intake of oxidized fats, and reduce the circulation of fats in your blood after a meal.

You must eat fewer fried foods, to be able to effectively lower your blood cholesterol.

Although, oxidized fats cannot be totally avoided, your body has the ability to prevent fat from being oxidized, and neutralizes fat that would have reacted with oxygen.

To be able to get your body to have this defense mechanism, your body needs a daily supply of antioxidants from your diets.

The following antioxidant nutrients with their food sources will help you get the best in having a healthy heart.

1. Vitamin A: Sources of vitamin A are beta-carotene, egg yolk, and liver.

2. Vitamin C: Sources include peppers, broccoli, citrus, melons, berries, and tropical fruits.

3. Vitamin E: Sources include nuts, wheat germ, seeds and their oils.

4. Beta-carotene: sources include sweet potatoes, apricots, paw-paw, and dark yellow and green vegetables.

5. Selenium: sources include: Red meat, whole grains, nuts, and sea foods.

6. Zinc: Sources include whole grains, oysters, liver, and sea foods.

You must avoid high fat ingredients, including butter, oil, cream, and sour cream. Also, avoid high fat foods like cheese, sausage, and avocado, and high fat cooking methods like broiling with butter, and frying.

Endeavor to watch your cholesterol level, by consuming less saturated fat, from foods like full fat yogurt, cheese, whole milk, and sour cream; and less Trans fat present in fried and processed foods. It is recommended to eat more of fish.

Avoid high oil and sodium diets, and make sure you cut down on these by eating steamed rice instead of fried Also, avoid egg rolls, fried dumplings, and higher fat diets like pork. In addition avoid deep fried chicken and fish.

This is so because there are many problems involved with fried food, as they are not good food for a healthy heart. If you desire a healthy heart, eat good foods as outlined above.

Proper Eating and Best Foods for Energy

Food is the fuel of our body craves and eating the right type of food is very important, in order that we may keep our body strong and full of energy. If you desire to loss weight, eating small amount of food, exercise regularly can be help you to achieve the goal, in addition to other things.

The following guide will help you get the best out of proper eating and best energy foods.

1. Consume the right type of food

Consume grains, fruits, and vegetables regularly. Also, make sure that you stay away from fried foods or fatty foods. Consume up to four or five small meals, rather than one or two large bowls.

Try not to miss or skip breakfast or other meals, so that your body system will function normally. Avoid junk foods, like cakes, sweets, and fast foods.

2. Eat high energy foods daily

Your stress level can be managed or reduced with regular and daily consumption of high energy foods. The following best high energy foods.

a. Oatmeal

Oatmeal is a source of fiber. Fiber has the ability to help your digestion, so that you body can have a steady flow of energy as carbohydrate enters into your blood system. Eating fiber means eating the right type of food.

b. Beans

Beans aid the problem of low iron deficiency which brings the problem of sluggishness. Beans is best eaten when prepared as soup.

c. Snack Banana

Bananas contain potassium, a mineral element that help in nerves and muscles normal functioning.

d. Green Spinach

Green spinach contains the magnesium mineral. Consuming spinach ensures that are taking in adequate levels of the mineral.

e. Strawberries

Strawberries can aid your body to absorb iron, because it contains vitamin C.

f. Soybean Products

Soybeans have many health benefits and contain calcium. It can be consume as soymilk, and other products.

g. Other high energy foods include tuna, whole grain bagels, and low-fat yogurt.

3. Drink water daily and regularly

Water is very important for our body's well-being. Water helps in digestion of food in the body, and keeps the body and skin in optimal conditions.

It is recommended that you take eight to ten glasses of water daily. You can start with 2 glasses of water, first thing in the morning.

Work out your proper eating and use of best foods for energy, for good health, physical fitness, and a better skin.

Beauty and Immunity Boosting Foods That Fight Aging

This article provides information about some beauty foods and immunity boosting foods that fight wrinkles smooth the skin, give healthy eyes, and drives cold and flu.

The following beauty foods are also able to build up the muscles and burn of fats in the body:

1. Sweet potatoes - Smooth skin

This vegetable is packed full with beauty boosting anti oxidant, called beta carotene. When you consume sweet potatoes, your body works on the beta carotene and convert it to vitamin A, which then keeps your skin to be silky smooth.

A serving of sweet potatoes provides a double dose of vitamin A needs and has much of beta carotene.

2. Blueberries - Fights wrinkles

The garnish, blueberries, in your morning oatmeal, can help to lower the signs of aging, with high antioxidant content, vitamin C and E in particular, which strengthens collagen formation by reducing harmful free radical damage.

3. Spinach - gives good eye health

It is reported that most people depended on spinach for muscle strength, and that eating spinach is a major reason why many people do not need eyeglasses.

Also, one cup of cooked spinach gives the highest amount of elements known for preventing vision loss among vegetables.

It is recommended that you add olive oil, garlic, and lemon juice, and cook for two minutes.

4. Mushrooms

It is recommended that you toss in mushrooms. Mushrooms, according to research, are said to contain Beta-glucan, a type of sugar, has potent antiviral and antibacterial properties.

5. Salmon

It is reported that salmon contain lean protein that fights diseases, and also has good fats that help strengthen cell membranes, which help to speed up any healing time.

6. Pumpkin and other Leafy vegetables

These vegetables contain chemical plant compounds that fight disease-causing free radicals.

7. Garlic

Garlic is a natural germ fighter. It is made up of an antibacterial compound. Research has it that this helps to stimulate white blood cells involved in immunity work. It is recommended that you take two raw gloves of garlic daily.

Foods and Supplements to Prevent and Improve Poor Eyesight

Your eyes respond to lifestyle and dietary changes, which may go along way to promote healthy eyesight or bring about poor eyesight. Foods and supplements have a role to play in preventing and improving poor eyesight.

As one continues to age, the eyes become less active, but foods and supplements can be used to prevent or improve them.

As you age, old sightedness, a type of farsighted that results from aging occurs. This type of farsightedness comes normally and gradually with age. With age, the crystalline lens of the eyes becomes less transparent, and tends to lose its elasticity.

The lens at this time fails to thicken properly and casts images behind instead of on the retina. Some persons at the age of forty and above begin to hold the newspaper farther and farther away, to be able to read it.

Damage to the eyes is often caused by environmental pollution, toxins, and poor diets deficient in essential nutrients. Damage is also caused by bye products of normal functioning of the body.

Eye diseases such as cataracts, glaucoma, and age-related eye degeneration, may occur as from age 40 and above.

Foods and supplements can help prevent and improve poor eyesight, because the eyes respond well to lifestyle changes and diets.

The following foods and supplements can help prevent and improve poor eyesight:

1. Eat Garlic and onions

These foods contain sulphur, which form glutathione. Glutathione protects the lens, and aids in the prevention of cataracts, experts say.

2. Add Bilberry to your Diet

This food helps strengthen capillaries in the eyes, improves blood circulation to the retina, and helps the production of a purple pigment that is used by the eye rods for night vision, experts say.

3. Eat Red Peppers and Tomatoes

These foods are also known to reduce the risk of cataracts. These foods contain good amounts of vitamin C.

4. Eat Yellow Vegetables, Carrot and deep Oranges

They contain beta-carotene, which help to reduce the risk of eye degeneration trouble due to age.

5. Eat Broccoli, Spinach, and Green vegetables

Experts say that they help to shield the eyes from ultra violet rays.

6. Daily Ingest Multivitamins and Antioxidants Supplements

You must daily take antioxidants and multivitamins supplements. These provide all the essential nutrients that are required by the eye for normal and optimal functioning, which may be missing in your diets.

They will aid the eye to receive normal blood circulation, nerve function, and general eye health.

How to Have a Healthy Blood Stream without Anemia

It is good to know about anemia and how to build up your blood system to be able to stay away from the dreaded disease called anemia.

Anemia is a blood disease, which is sometimes call ' thin blood '. There are many kinds of anemia, but the common types are iron deficiency anemia and pernicious anemia.

Some kind of anemia may result from the destruction of too many red blood cells or the loss of too many red blood cells through direct or hidden kind of bleeding.

The more common forms of anemia are caused by a failure of the blood forming system, located at the bone marrow, to manufacture adequate or the right type of red blood cells. This failure is usually because of the lack of iron and other essential nutrients in the diet.

Anemia symptoms include a) pale skin and mucous membranes, b) loss of appetite, c) easy fatigue, d) low energy, e) shortness of breath, f) palpitation of the heart, and g) general weakness.

In onset of pernicious anemia, symptom includes, numbness, tingling, and needles-and-pins sensations in the arms and legs. In addition the tongue may be sore and smooth.

You can enable your blood stream to begin to flow strongly and smoothly, by starting to revitalize your blood. To do this effectively, you need iron and copper. Wheat germ, molasses, and liver are the best sources of iron and copper.

Plan to begin consuming liver once or twice a week, including wheat germ and molasses without sulphur, in your day to day eating or diets.

Inadequate or unbalanced diets lacking in iron, copper, proteins, and vitamin B, results in marginal anemia, a situation where the body cannot produce enough healthy blood cells, to maintain a healthy blood stream. All ages may have a common complaint about this type of anemia.

The red cells contain more protein than iron, this makes protein of necessity. You also need all the essential amino acid for the optimal building of your blood.

Women are more vulnerable to anemia condition than men, because that lose blood on a monthly basis. They therefore net properly handle the problem of anemia.

It is possible to easily correct an anemic situation or condition, when your diet contain optimal amounts of complete protein, made available through milk, meat, eggs, wheat germ and brewer's yeast.

The formation of a healthy blood must obtain all of vitamin B, namely thiamine, niacin, folic acid, etc. It is known that lack of folic acid and vitamin B12, seem to be a cause of anemic condition, called pernicious anemia.

Necessity of Vitamins and Supplements for Healthy Living

Vitamins are organic substances produced from plants and some animal sources. For an individual to remain healthy and grow normally, vitamins are required in very small quantities.

Lack of the necessary amounts, may bring about a vitamin deficiency disease, called a vitaminosis. Examples of such diseases include beriberi, rickets, scurvy, and pellagra.

Vitamin supplements are sometimes clearly necessary, whenever the dietary intake of vitamins is inadequate. Multivitamins plus minerals in capsule or tablet form, taken once a day goes along way to fortify your diet. A good mixed diet of common foods, will supply all the vitamins needed.

But because a good mixed diet of common foods, including protective foods, may be lacking, or if present, may be destroyed through cooking, there is therefore the need for a multivitamins plus minerals capsule or tablets to be taken daily.

Sometimes this problem occurs when on a low-calorie reducing diet, after surgical operation, during pregnancy, and during a serious illness.

Vitamin deficiency are mostly of multiple rather than single in a particular diet, it is therefore necessary to take vitamin supplements prescribed to treat certain diseases and conditions, because, they supply a balance of all vitamins.

It is now recommended that a mixed diet should be taken, so that all the vitamins will be present. In considering a mixed diet, only a few vitamins should be taken seriously. This is so because, when these few vitamins are present, others also become present.

These vitamins of importance are vitamin A, C, D, and three members of vitamin B complex (thiamine, niacin, and riboflavin).

Vitamin A (retinol)

Vitamin A is essential to growth and development. It maintains the normal functioning of the cells lining the throat and the eyelids. It is needed for normal night vision.

Vitamin A aids growth and tooth formation. If absent or deficient, or lacking, results in night blindness- seeing poorly in the dim light. It reduces resistance to colds and other throat and eye infections. Continued shortage of vitamin A may result in blindness.

Sources of vitamin A are liver, kidneys, whole milk, butter, eggs, and tomatoes, all green and yellow vegetables (carrots, corn, and sweet potatoes).

These yellow vegetables contain carotene, a substance from which vitamin A is produced. Palm oil is rich in carotene. A mixed diet containing the above sources is very necessary for good health.

Vitamin B complex comprises of a large number of water soluble vitamins, including thiamine, riboflavin, niacin, folic acid, etc.

Thiamine is essential for utilization of carbohydrates, normal appetite, and function of the digestive tract. Severe deficiency results in beriberi- a serious nervous disorder.

Sources of thiamine are whole grains, meat, fish, and vegetables. Proper cooking is required in order not to destroy it.

Riboflavin is essential for growth, health, and cell respiration. It helps to maintain healthy skin and proper coordination of muscles. Deficiency results in stunted growth, scaly, sore skin and eye diseases.

The vitamin is found in yeast, liver, kidneys, milk, eggs, and green vegetables.

Niacin is needed for proper use of carbohydrates in the body. It is also called pellagra-preventive vitamin. Deficiency results in skin rash, stomach upset, paralysis and mental disorders.

Sources are garden vegetables, lean meat, liver, eggs, and yeast.

Vitamin C (ascorbic acid)

This vitamin is necessary in building and maintaining well-developed blood vessels and gums. It also helps to prevent infections. Deficiency causes blood vessels to break down, and a serious disease called scurvy develops (swelling of the tongues and bleeding of the gums and joints).

Best sources are all the citrus fruits (orange, lime, lemon, grapefruit, and tangerine), tomatoes, green peppers, cabbage, and uncooked leafy vegetables such as lettuce.

Vitamin D (calciferol)

Vitamin D is also called the Sunshine Vitamin. It can be manufactured in the skin. Lack of vitamin D in the body results in rickets (faulty growth of bones and teeth in children). This may cause deformed chest and bow legs.

Sources found are liver, fish liver oil, milk, and eggs.

It is better to fortify your diet with a multiple vitamins plus minerals capsule or tablets, in case the inability to provide a mixed diet containing all the vitamins and minerals or should some be destroyed during cooking.

B. Exercise and Physical Fitness

We have seen already that physical activity or exercise is very important in physical fitness and wellness. Let's look further.

Basic Principles of Exercises

There are various basic exercise principles to help you handle different components of your workout or fitness goals.

An effective exercise or fitness program can be ensured when basic principles of exercise are adhered to. These exercise principles are stated as follows:

Frequency

Your physical fitness or exercise goals can be achieved with effectiveness when you exercise often or regularly. You are expected to exercise for at least five times a week. Ensure that you keep being regular to avoid doing harm to your exercise goals.

You can add more days of a particular type of exercise, if expected body improvements are no more seen. So, how often do you exercise?

Balance

Plan your exercise program to ensure a balance of activities for your fitness. Your exercise activities should take care of muscle strength, muscle endurance, flexibility, body composition, and aerobic or cardio-respiratory components of physical fitness.

Doing so will create a balance and not harm to any of the components of physical fitness.

Intensity

In your exercise program you need to start from less swift or less hard to swift or hard. That is from low intensity to high intensity.

Also, you need to make sure that your duration of exercise be increased gradually, to help you achieve those fitness goals of yours. Therefore how hard you exercise matters.

Variety

Endeavor to engage in different types of exercises or physical activities. This will enable you to exercise without becoming bored by creating a motivation force to carry on. You will also experience likeness to the various varieties of activities.

The particular type of exercise you are involved in matters, in terms of training effect in line with your physical fitness goal.

Different types of exercises exist, such as running, jogging, bicycling, walking, and swimming. If body improvement is no longer seen in one exercise, do the other activity.

Recovery

You need a rest period or less rigorous activity or training. Ensure that you alternate days for physical activity involving muscular endurance and muscular strength components of physical fitness.

Never work the same muscles two days in a row, this will enable your body to have enough time to rest and recover. You need at least a day of rest between strength training workouts.

Specificity

Your exercise training should be motivated by set goals that are specific in nature rather than broad. Is it to shed some weight, build up muscles, or the actual attainment of physical fitness? Endeavor to engage in a type of exercise that can enable you achieve a specific goal.

Overload

As you exercise towards your specific goals in each exercise session, each work load should exceed that of the normal demanded by your body, in order to achieve the effectiveness expected.

You need to progressively increase the intensity, frequency, and time of your training. Do try different types of exercise.

Time

This involves how long you exercise in an exercise session. If you are no more seeing changes or improvement in your fitness program, there is need to add few minutes to your usual training or workout time to get require training effect.

The above basic exercise principles are linked to one another and must be seriously taken into consideration for your success in any exercise program

Boost Your Health with Regular Exercise

Expert researches and studies, say that regular exercise is very important, and has health benefits. The following health benefits of exercise would help you get the best out of regular exercise.

1. Regular exercise improves the quality and duration of sleep.

Your sleep becomes sweet with regular exercise. The inability to sleep would be taken away. When you wake up, you would not experience fatigue. You would have a better night rest, wake up strong, and active.

2. Regular exercise reduces anxiety and depression.

Vigorous exercise done regularly reduces feelings of anger, depression, and confusion.

It takes you to a high point, whereby anxiety diminishes, depression vanishes, and you put on a feeling of good health. Exercise is known to improve your mood, leaving no room for depression moods.

To manage anxiety, get regular exercise, such as bicycle riding, jogging, and brisk walking around. Researches found that exercising for 20 to one hour, three times a week, diminishes depression.

3. Regular exercise refreshes, invigorates, and improves health.

Your blood flow would improve. Oxygen and nutrients supply to your brain improves, thereby giving you mental alertness, and ability to think better.

4. Regular exercise relieves stress.

Jogging, swimming, and brisk walking can help relief stress and give you a positive outlook and life. You become physically fit, emotionally sound, and mentally alert.

Stress breaks down your body's immune system and makes you vulnerable to common infections like common colds, etc, and memory impairment.

5. Regular exercise helps boost your sense of self-worth.

Engaging in exercises that stretch and strengthen you, makes you feel better and able to face the world.

6. Regular exercise gives your mind needed time out from daily responsibility and duties.

7. Regular exercise strengthens your bones, and opens your chest.

Your joints, legs, hands, bones, spines, and chest, become strengthened as you engage in exercise. Your posture would improve.

Your chest would open, allowing you to have deep regular breathing that your body needs.

8. Regular exercise takes pains away.

Pains that often come with waking up in the morning, and the weakness that follow, would go with regular exercise.

9. Regular exercise would help you cut down on excess weight, and give you that fitness and health you need.

10. Regular exercise imparts and impacts vigor, youthfulness, and beauty in your look and life.

With the above benefits of regular exercise, in mind, there is need to discipline yourself and engage in regular exercise on a daily basis, to be able to reap the benefits that follow.

Risks Associated with Exercise

Exercise is very beneficial, yet there arises risks that ranges from minor to serious and even sudden death. These risks are caused by ignorance and wrong approaches or methods.

These risks are actually warning or danger signs that cause the exercise to be counterproductive, instead of achieving your physical fitness set goals.

Time taken up by exercise may not be considered as exercise risk, if your exercise is done on scheduled, and never becomes counterproductive in any way.

If exercise is carried out in a wrong way or at a wrong time, exercise risks or danger signs will arise.

Such exercise risks include: Severe Fatigue, Muscle Cramps, and Severe Chest

Pain, Loss of Concentration, Sleeplessness, Fainting Spells, Ringing in the Ears, Headaches, Gasping for Breath, Dehydration, Soreness, Stiffness, overheating, Injury, or even Sudden Death.

Sudden Death

Some people who go for paramilitary interviews, drop death when engaged while running. This may be caused by a major factor called coronary heart disease.

How to Avoid Risks of Exercise

Risks of exercise can be avoided by taking heed to the following tips:

You must wear Comfortable Clothes and socks, Wear Supportive Shoes, Consult your Doctor or Trainer, Stay Hydrated, Avoid Exercising in Hot

Weather, vary activities, avoid exercising when ill, stop when fatigued, and progressing gradually.

Other measures to avoid risks of exercise include: avoiding rugged terrain, avoid falling activities, do exercises that suit you, avoid over-rigorous activities, avoid exercising on a full stomach, and always begin and end with warm-up and cool down.

Exercising for Physical Fitness

Physical fitness involves a number of things of which exercise has to be considered. The following tips would help you become physically fit, as you put them into practice:

Exercise aims at maintaining and giving fitness, health, strong bones, weight loss and a general well-being. When exercise is done properly, in addition to rest, sleep, and good diet, it brings desired goals.

Exercise comes in different forms, such as jogging, swimming, bicycle riding, weight lifting, walking, jump rope type, etc.

All categories of persons are expected to perform one exercise or the other based on their state of health. Some persons who are diabetic need to seek the approval of a medical doctor for help in exercising, to avoid injury.

Exercise has been proved through research to give great benefits to the body, such as:

i. Putting up strong bones

ii. Gives a healthy weight, by removing excess fat in the body

iii. Reduction in the risk of some illnesses like diabetes, hypertension, and cancer;

iv. Exercise is shown to improve one's self-worth and much more, as we have already discussed.

When one is able to go on with the activities of the day without stress, such can say fitness is into play. At this time the body is strong and able to carry out various activities, and being immune to most infections, like common cold.

Physical fitness comes to stay when such factors like muscle strength, flexibility, muscle endurance, body composition, and cardio-respiratory endurance comes into play.

Exercise is so important that all need to have it on a daily basis, to be able to significantly improve their quality of life.

As a rule, it is recommended that one has to get exercise for 15 – 30 minutes at a time, without stopping, to be able to profit optimally.

You must exercise sufficiently to increase your pulse rate to about two third your maximum heart rate. This level must also be maintained for 15-30 minutes without stopping.

However, when stopping, one should observe a cooling down period, and not just to stop abruptly. It can be dangerous, when the heart is beating heavily.

When about to stop abruptly, slow down your speed or heart beat rate, by slowing down the activity or exercise.

Research has shown that even brisk walking alone can still be beneficial, and may add to one's life span.

Exercising outdoors by brisk walking to stretch out one's legs, at least once a week, is shown to be beneficial, when discipline is taken seriously.

Best Exercise for fitness and Health

Exercise is very important for the human body. Exercise is known to dissolve many disorders of the body. This happens when one engages in vigorous exercise.

As you continue in the degree of your exercise, infections like common colds subside, diseases that are degenerative in nature disappear, life quality improves, and life span increases.

To understand which exercise is best for fitness and health, consider the following points:

1. Competitive sports are not the best exercises for certain ages.

Competitive sports should remain with the youths. But it comes to time when the body really needs exercise, when one has attained the age of 35 and above, this is when exercise is beneficial and required.

At this time, you should start exercising for better life. This is because; your health would begin to deteriorate during this time, if you refuse to give attention to exercise.

This deterioration in health usually occurs because you are no more involved competitive sports, and because you are aging.

2. Characteristics of Best Exercise.

Best exercise should be characterized by vigorous workouts and should be non-violent. For example, running and jogging. You must maintain a high level of athletic training, to make running and jogging safe.

If you have no training, limit yourself to non-violent exercises like walking, and then get training for vigorous exercises, for your improve quality of life.

3. Non-Competitive Sports or Best Exercise.

You must get training or learn the sport that is non-competitive. This is sport that can be enjoyed alone. Start out with 30 minutes daily, and move on to about one hour daily. Spend this time in vigorous exercise outdoor.

Also, spend another 30 minutes to about one hour daily indoor, in such activities that require muscular energy to be expended.

Your physical condition and fitness would be better when you get involved in these vigorous exercises.

4. Why you must Exercise Vigorously

a. This type of exercise is the secret behind your having vigor, youthfulness, and beauty. Just take your exercise seriously. Start jogging in the morning and in the evening, if you are chanced, and reap the benefits.

b. This type of exercise would keep you in good shape and active too.

Make exercise, part of your daily routine activity.

c. If you are a beginner in exercise, you may get the services of a trainer or professional to supervise what you do. That means you pay to get the best result. You can also learn as you go along daily.

d. You would become alert, fit, and healthy as you exercise.

 Exercise would help you cut down and maintain your weight. If you fail to exercise, you would start putting on weight.

e. Get involved also with swimming.

When you swim, you exercise some major muscles of your body. Some persons classify swimming as their number one exercise.

To stay fit, healthy, and happy, daily give yourself a dose of vigorous exercise that you enjoy doing.

How to Stay Healthy with Home Workout Routines

There is need to know how to stay healthy with home workout routines.

Staying healthy and fit can be achieved even when one makes use of home work out routines, in the absence of time to go to the gym.

With concentration and discipline, home workout routines can help you stay in shape and have that desirable body you need, and here is how.

Plan Time for Workout

Plan your time of regular workouts if you can or try to engage in workouts at least 3 to 5 times weekly. Avoid distractions by cutting off any means of communication, such as silencing your phones.

Plan a Full Body Workout

Plan a full body workout instead of aiming at body parts. Add variations to your exercises and never perform same exercises daily to avoid boredom and discontinuation of workout program.

Get Instant Energy before Workout

Eat carbohydrates that give instant energy before a workout. You can also make use of instant glucose D for instant energy.

Get Home Workout Equipment and Start

Simple and easy to use workout equipment to make use of includes, stretch bands, jump ropes, medicine balls or exercise balls, etc.

You need to warm up before you start a stretching routine at the end of your workout to prevent muscles soreness and keep you limber at best for the next day.

Following a good diet regime is also important in achieving desired results to avoid working out without results.

Getting results entails that you follow a workout plan of cardiovascular exercise plus diet and sticking to it for about 8 to 10 weeks. This will enable you to stay motivated and continue without stopping.

Engage in Sample Home Workout Routines

Home workout routines abound to help you stay healthy and fit. The following sample home workout routines can help you begin and stay healthy at home without going to a gym:

Boxing and kicking

These can be done without any equipment, by just boxing and kicking the air at any spacious part of your apartment. You can also turn your right leg outward and inward and then kick the air. Do same for the left leg immediately after the right leg.

Pushups and Sit-ups Routines:

Push-up Routine

You can go about this as follows: Lie with face down on the ground, keep hands at shoulder width apart directly begin the shoulder, and keep your body completely straight from head to toes or to knees(when you need to reduce difficulty or stress).

If you keep knees to the ground, you need to cross your legs at the ankles.

Start pushing your body up and down bending your elbow joints to bring about motion. You can do up to five to ten or more push-ups at a time depending on your fitness ability. Rest and then do more one or two sets of push-ups.

Sit-up Routine

Lie down flat on the ground or floor with your back and knees bent, with feet kept at six inches above the ground and your hands behind your head or resting on the floor close to your hips. Lift your knees towards your chest, while breathing in slowly, until your bottom is off the floor.

Now slowly return your legs to starting position while breathing out slowly.

Repeat this motion for five or more times, rest for a short while before doing again. You should repeat set two or more times for maximum benefit.

Crunch and Leg Raises

Crunches:

Lie on your back with your hands behind your head and feet in the air making your thighs vertical. Keep your chin off your chest and keep your elbows wide, exhale and lift your shoulders off the floor.

Leg Raise:

Lie face up on the ground with your hands behind your head. Bring your body up in crunch position and hold at the top. Keep your legs straight, and draw your belly button in towards your spine as you exhale.

Curl your tailbone under and roll up the spine as if you were trying to bring your knees to your head. Return slowly to start position.

Exercise Ball Workout

Ball exercises require little and inexpensive equipment. In performing the majority of ball exercises you only need to buy an exercise ball.

In addition, you may add a pair of dumb bells or workout bench. You can sit on the exercise ball; fall slightly on it with your back, etc.

Exercise Band Workout for Stretching Routines

Band exercises are widely used for general strength and conditioning and rehabilitation or injury prevention.

Band exercises can help condition cardiovascular system as well as strengthening specific muscle groups.

One way of performing exercise band is to lie on the floor and loop band around the right foot, grabbing onto the bands to create tension. Straighten the right leg as much as possible while keeping the left leg bent on the floor.

Next, slowly pull the right leg towards you, stretching the back of the leg.

Maintain the exercise for 10 to 30 seconds and exchange to the other side.

Jump Rope

Use this to shed weight. This can be used as a warm up routine too.

How to Develop a Regular Exercise Routine

We here describe how to develop a regular exercise routine, on a daily basis, so as to reap the enormous benefits that exercising provides.

The following guide would enable you become consistent in your workout routines, and therefore make a regular habit.

Plan Workouts to Engage in Weekly

Those who fail to plan, plan to fail, is a known saying. So, plan well before you start exercising. Planning weekly helps in giving you what type of workout routines to engage in throughout each week.

Your weekly exercise plan may depend on your fitness and health goals.

Are you exercising to build muscles, burn fat, or for general health? Your workout routines would differ accordingly.

Your plan may be: Sunday-Boxing and kicking the air, Monday – Exercise ball workout, Wednesday – crunch and leg raises, etc.

Progress Slowly in your Weekly Workouts

As a beginner, never crowd your week with too many workout routines, so as not to get frustrated, and made to quit. You can do two or three workout routines in two or three days of a week.

Set Goals to Help Determine your Success

Your set goals would help you know what you actually want. You may be exercising to build muscles or for weight loss, your goals would help determine your success.

Make it a Habit to Exercise in the Morning

Exercising early in the morning would help you become consistent and thereby make it a regular habit.

It is in the morning you may have the time to do your set workout routines, so endeavor to do so.

Evaluate your Goals and Seriousness Weekly

You must evaluate yourself weekly to see whether you are following through and performing your weekly workout routines or if your goals are being met.

Exercising regularly would help you meet your target goals, whether fitness or health. So, start now and become consistent as you follow the above guide on how to develop a regular exercise routine.

How to Focus on an Exercise Routine

There are tips how to focus on an exercise routine with the aim of helping you to achieve your set goals for fitness and health. These tips include:

Focus on Set Goals

Never be over concern with your weight measurement at the beginning, but rather focus on your set goals.

Therefore you need to put the weighing scales out of your exercise routine area, to avoid the temptation of being over concern on getting immediate results as you turn often to see the numbers on the scale.

This can cause you to lose focus of your target or set goals, due to discouragement from the results.

Keep a Measurement Tape Nearby

You to keep a chart of your progress or success, by keeping a measurement tape nearby for taking measurements of your waist, hips, chest, thighs, and upper arms.

You can take measurements every three weeks and charting the measurements, as you exercise

Do Things you Love Doing

As you carryout your exercise routine, do the things you love. Get involved in volunteer services, buy things you love, read good things you love.

You can also listen to good music, even while carrying out your exercise routine or after.

Take pictures now and then to see the differences in weight gain, weight loss, or whatever your set goals are.

Have a Merry Heart While Exercising

Make contact with people and rejoice and be happy. Free your heart from worry and anxiety. Meet often with your love ones and spouse, to share or chat with them.

Be Nice to yourself

Give yourself some nice treatment, as you see your progress and success. You need to give time to rest well, travel, care for your body, and check up on your physical and spiritual health.

Keeping focused on exercise routine as outlined above would help you achieve your set goals on weight loss, weight gain, or whatever the goals may be. Start slowly and progress towards your goals and success.

Ways to Get in Shape through Daily Exercise

Here comes information on ways to get in shape through a regular program of daily exercise.

Daily exercise is necessary for you to be productive, lively, agile, and healthy.

So, daily move your whole body for energy needed, by finding and abiding to certain exercises you cherish and enjoy. The following guides would do you good:

Select activities you enjoy partaking throughout the year.

Activities abound that can change your life. So, try and find activities that you can engage in throughout the year, like swimming and skiing in their proper season. Participate in activities that are enriching and live giving.

Set Goals for Exercise

Set exercise goals for long term and short term. Your goal can be to engage in jogging every day and to walk briskly every day.

Your reasons for exercising can also be stated to help you stay focused. With time your goal of getting in shape through exercise shall be attained.

Let your muscles make your strong

You can exercise outdoors and indoors to keep fit and get in shape. But you can still do so indoors by using the sitting room or staircase to jog, jump, lift weights, stretching your body and run around, etc.

Choose an appropriate time for your exercise

You can get in shape through exercise by keeping to the right time to undertake exercise daily.

Chose a time that you will be free from distraction from other activities that may try to rob you of your exercise. Once this is done, stick to it. It may be 7.00am or 6.00am or as desired.

Join a fitness class to get monitored

A fitness class will help put you on a different footing altogether, where you get the best from trained personnel.

Exercise with others

Exercising with others will help you learn from those who know more than you and also get the excitement of togetherness.

As you exercise on a daily basis and regularly, you will definitely get in shape, and look healthy.

Methods or Ways to Lose Weight

Here are the top most and easy methods of reducing weight, without stress or unnecessary expenditure.

Getting on with life and having a balanced diet on a daily basis is the desire for many. Living without this, is the result of most people being over-weight.

Below are tested methods or tips in which appreciable results have been obtain in shedding away unwanted weight gain.

1. Do not skip breakfast.

Make sure that you get up early enough each day, so as not to miss your daily breakfast.

This is very important because breakfast is both good for your health and getting rid of excess weight. Breakfast would help your body to accept food throughout the day.

Make sure you start your breakfast with some high fiber and low starch fruits. You may decide to eat fruits all through the day, but do not forget to start that with breakfast.

2. Drink About 8 - 10 Glasses of Water Daily.

You can become used to this by starting out first thing in the morning. You can take 2 glasses immediately after waking from sleep, first thing in the morning before eating food.

This can help create an awareness of the need to make up the remaining glasses through the day. Water is not bitter, so you must try and drink it first thing in the morning.

3. Do Physical Exercise Daily and Regularly

Exercise can help you reduce weight and also maintain it. When you wake up stretch your hands, legs, neck, and body. Breathe in and out for about five minutes at a time.

You can also do some work up like weight lifting, jogging, jumping, etc This should be done daily and regularly in the morning.

4. Avoid Junk Food.

Make sure that you avoid these foods that are called fast foods and such others like sweets, cakes, fried foods, and snacks.

Eat much of fruits. Your diet should contain more of fruits than carbohydrates. Get oranges, melons, grapes, etc.

5. Eat Enough Of Vegetables Daily.

You need vegetables to get enough fiber in your diet. If you have stop eating vegetables daily, start doing so regularly. You can look out in cookery books for their recipes and enjoy yourself.

Your weight loss is very important for having a healthy body and living a long life, so get involved in the necessary methods and shed that extra weight.

Eight simple Ways to flatten your tummy and look younger

Living a life with a bloated tummy portrays one as having no knowledge of what to do, in order to avoid, flatten, or control one's stomach.

Though many things may result in a bloated tummy, there are simple ways in which one can use to flatten his or her stomach, in order to remain or look younger. These simple ways are as follows:

1. Drink 8 - 10 Glasses of Water Daily.

Drinking lots of water daily would help to flush your system of clogs and impurities. So, drink lots of water daily, up to 8 - 10 glasses.

Drinking much water daily, would make you to eat less food. This is so because; the water would reduce hunger pangs, which would have caused you to eat much.

Much water helps in digestion, thereby removing the problem of a bloated tummy. Lots of water taken daily would help to flush any bloating your experience.

2. Avoid or Stop the intake of Alcohol.

Alcohol is dangerous to your health. Medical report say that alcohol causes bloating of tummy, due to its ability to cause the accumulation of fat in the stomach, by raising cortisol levels in the body. Alcohol is also known to dehydrate the body, leaving patches of bloats in tummy.

3. Consume More Fiber Daily.

Fiber in your diets would help prevent bloating due to constipation. Fiber diets also help to reduce your weight, including tummy weight gain.

Cut down your intake of carbohydrates, such as white bread and white rice. To get fiber you need, take vegetables, fruits, brown, and whole wheat bread.

4. Eat Balanced and Small Portions of Food or Meals.

Eat small portions of food or meals throughout the day, than eating 2 – 3 big portions. Smaller portions eaten many times a day would help digestion to take place faster, to avoid giving your tummy a bloated look.

Eat healthy snacks like almonds every morning and night, which help in burning fat, and sometimes just take desserts, all these helps to flatten your tummy.

Consume calcium diets or take it as a daily supplement of 1000mg to 1200mg.

This would help keep your bones strong, and avoid fractured bones that cause slump looks. Avoid much intake of whole milk, it causes bloating of the tummy.

5. Engage in Daily Regular Exercise.

Exercise for 30 minutes to one hour indoors and 30 minutes to one hour outdoor daily or five times a week. This can be done in small amount of time per moment. Go jogging, swimming, brisk walking, and running.

Do weight lifting, bench press to build your chest, and practice perfect posture exercises. Also, always sit and stand straight. Never slump when sitting down. Be active daily.

Exercise would help your system to be able to burn fat faster, thereby eliminating the problem of a bloated tummy.

6. Do Deep Breathing Daily.

Make sure that you do deep breathing for about 5 minutes daily. This should involve breathing from your abdomen, and not from your chest. So, try to take the deep breath from your lower abdomen. This would help to pull your tummy back and help the burning of fat.

7. Avoid or Manage Your Stressful Life.

Medical report say that too much of stress results in increases in levels of a hormone, called cortisol levels, thus enabling fat to be sent to the stomach.

You must manage stress appropriately. Learn to rest well and eliminate stressful activities.

8. Quit or Stop Smoking.

As in stress, smoking is also reported to raise levels of cortisol. This causes smokers to have increases in abdominal fat, thus a bloated tummy.

As you seek to flatten your tummy, do not give up easily, just follow the above tips, and you shall get a flattened tummy that gives you fitness and a younger look you desire.

4. Basic Exercises for Physical Fitness

There are two types of exercise. These are aerobic and anaerobic exercises.

The exercise type that you perform depends on your goals, health and fitness status, and preferences. Aerobic means with oxygen, and anaerobic means without oxygen.

Aerobic Exercises

Aerobic exercise is any physical activity of lower intensity. Aerobic exercise includes lower intensity activities undertaken for longer periods of time.

Examples are walking, long slow runs, rowing, and cycling requires a great deal of oxygen to generate the energy needed for prolonged exercise.

i. Brisk Walking

Of all the ways to get and stay fit, walking is the easiest, safest and cheapest.

It can also be a lot of fun, with attainable goals. Here are some suggestions to help you get the most out of your walking workouts.

You want to be comfortable while you walk. Shoes that are specially designed for walking have flexible soles and stiff heel counters to prevent side-to-side motion.

But for normal terrain, almost any comfortable, cushioned, lightweight, low-heeled shoes will do just fine. It's best to avoid stiff soled shoes that don't bend.

Excellent walking workouts include:

Must do it daily

You should walk briskly for at least half an hour every day; try more frequent, shorter walks, than one single walk of half an hour.

Other walking workouts are counting your steps when you do walk to see if you have done much walking, using the staircase, swinging your arms as you walk, climbing hills, and experiencing something else.

ii. Stretching

Stretching is a type of exercise involving the deliberate flexing of specific muscles or muscle group, meant to improve the muscle and achieve proper muscle tone. Passive stretching daily is good for your fitness.

iii. Running and Jogging

This can be done indoor or outdoor, at short distances or longer.

iv. Natural Deep Breathing

Natural deep breathing is highly required for a good functioning of the body and fitness.

How to Perform Natural Deep Breathing Exercise

Natural deep breathing improves health. Here are given ways of properly engaging in natural deep breathing.

To benefit from natural deep breathing, follow the steps below:

1. Know The Benefits Of Deep Breathing.

If you have not read my article on health benefits of deep breathing, you can check it out after, but here is a brief list that have been established by doctors and experts in natural deep breathing:

a. Through deep breathing the diaphragm moves downward and massages the stomach, liver, and other organs below it. Also, when it moves upwards, it massages the heart.

b. The upward and downward movement of the diaphragm detoxifies your inner organs and promotes blood flow.

c. Deep Breathing helps to pump the lymph more efficiently through the lymphatic system, which is part of our immune system.

d. Natural deep breathing helps in reducing stress in our lives.

e. Natural deep breathing improves our general health.

f. Deep breathing increases vitality, promotes relaxation and prolongs longevity

2. How to Perform Natural Deep Breathing

The technique of natural deep breathing is easy to understand. When you must have understood the technique, you can then begin to benefit from natural deep breathing.

To understand and do the exercise, follow the tips below:

i. Start your fitness exercise with natural deep breathing

ii. Seek a quiet and comfortable place that is void of distraction.

iii. Lie down, sit down, or stand.

Just take a posture that is comfortable to you.

iv. Avoid tension and negative emotions

Get your mind and muscles in a state of relaxation, to avoid having shallow breathing.

v. Inhale slowly and deeply, right from your lower abdomen, through your nostrils.

vi. Hold the breath while counting silently and slowly to 10 or just a count of 10 seconds.

vii. Exhale deeply with your mouth and nostrils open.

Make sure that you empty your lungs completely during this time.

viii. As you exhale, count to 5 or to a period of 5 seconds.

ix. Do or repeat the exercise for about 5 minutes or more, as stated above.

Remember to avoid distractions during this time, by concentrating your mind and physical being to the exercise only.

x. You must carryout this practice on a daily basis and regularly.

The above process is what you need to start enjoying and reaping the manifold health benefits of natural deep breathing.

Get your improved vitality and longevity through natural deep breathing.

Health Benefits of Natural Deep Breathing Exercise

Many experts in deep breathing exercise agree that there are numerous benefits that follow those who engage in deep breathing exercise.

Deep breathing has immense benefits to your health and has much effect in promoting longevity or life span.

Once the routine of deep breathing is started and continued, you would begin to reap immense benefits from its exercise.

The following stated benefits which experts in deep breathing have researched and acclaimed, would help you understand its importance and need for you to engage in the exercise:

1. Relaxation of Bowels

Deep breathing helps to relax your bowels. When trying to move your bowels in the toilet, deep breathing would enable you do so easily. While sitting on the toilet bowl, do deep breathing and your bowels would move.

2. Stress Reliever

Deep breathing relieves stress. Stress is injurious to health. Usually, the gross activities of a day, coupled with other factors, can bring about stress. But deep breathing works on your system, making it possible for you to be free from stress or less prone to stress.

3. Improves and Increases Oxygen Delivery and Supply to Body Organs

Deep breathing from the tummy helps provide an optimal supply of oxygen to all your body organs.

When deep breathing is routinely done, it both improves and increases delivery and level of oxygen supplied to body organs. This enables your system to do better.

4. Improves the Detoxification of body Organs and Cleanses the Body

Deep breathing, when done regularly, helps in the improvement of detoxification of body organs. When harmful poisons or toxins accumulate in the body, they cause harm. But deep breathing helps in the elimination of these toxins, and thus cleanses the body.

5. Deep Breathing Releases you from Anxiety

Deep breathing would help clear every clog in your mind, giving you a focused life, and thus releasing and relieving you from anxiety. Anxiety is dangerous to your health, and can cause many health problems and diseases.

6. Deep Breathing Promotes your Well-being

Deep breathing helps your system to release certain hormones that help to give you a sense of good health and well-being, relaxing your muscles. Thus, you get relief from muscle tension and pain.

7. Deep breathing improves your Physical and Mental Health

Your physical well-being is bound to improve as you engage in regular deep breathing. Also, your mental alertness improves, making it possible for you to be able to do what you could not do before.

8. Deep Breathing Helps to Lower your Blood Pressure

High blood pressure is that which many dread. With routine and regular deep breathing exercises, your blood pressure becomes lowered. Thus, bring your blood pressure to an approved level.

The key to success in deep breathing is regular and routine exercise. When you learn the ropes of deep breathing, apply them, and you shall reap all the above benefits.

iv. Swimming

Swimming is a water base exercise for health and fitness. A 30 minute swimming exercise for one or three days per week is good for fitness.

v. Bicycling

This can be done with bicycle upside down (without equipment) or with fixed or mobile bicycle.

How to Use Exercise Bicycle to Improve Fitness

We here present guides on how to raise or improve fitness with bicycle exercise.

Bicycle exercise can help meet your fitness goal. Your fitness level can be transformed with the use of bicycle exercise. This type of exercise can help to warm up your entire body, especially the heart.

So, biking is a good cardiovascular exercise for the development of a good heart. You need to consider biking in your fitness goal.

Make use of the following steps to better your fitness with bicycle exercise:

Check your Heart Rate at Rest

Before starting the biking exercise, you need to check your heart rate at rest, to help you compare that with heart rate during biking.

Use Biking Exercise to warm up your Body

Make use biking exercise to warm up your entire body in order to raise your fitness level.

You should also use some minutes biking as a warm up for the biking exercise, especially where competition is involved and when engaging in other cardiovascular exercises.

Maintain a Healthy Heart Rate Levels due to Age

After warming up, engage in full biking to better your fitness. While biking, take or check your heart rate using the heart rate monitor on the exercise bike or other means, to enable you maintain a healthy heart rate level suitable for your age.

Improve Fitness Using Different Routines

While biking, you need to make use of different bike routines to help you achieve your fitness goal. You need to carryout fat burning exercise and cardiovascular biking exercise, to raise your fitness level.

Exercise on Elevations for Improved heart Rate

Biking on elevations must be included during exercise biking. Biking hills or elevation will help you improve your heart rate and thus improve your fitness level.

Intensify your Biking for Better Fitness

Biking at low levels of intensity will not help you much with the exercise bike.

But for improved or better fitness level, there is the need to raise your biking intensity, in such a way as to achieve your goal.

Add Skills to your Biking for Improved Fitness

When your biking experience involves added skills, you are bound to enjoy your exercise, and at the same time help in improving your fitness level.

Added skills in biking will usually go with vigorous exercise, which is a sure way for better fitness level.

You need to develop skills and experience in exercise biking to enable you gain your best and achieve your fitness goal.

vi. Face and Body Massage

You can use your physical hands to massage your face or body. A machine can be used for body massage.

Anaerobic Exercises

Anaerobic means without oxygen. It is a short lasting, high intensity exercise or activity, that body demand for oxygen is greater than the oxygen supply present.

Examples of anaerobic exercise include weight lifting, sprinting, and jumping.

i. Weight Training or Weight Lifting Exercise

As a measure to keep fit, may decide to undertake a strength or weight lifting program. Whatever your goals, lean muscle gain, strength, fitness, or weight reduction, you can start out and get your decide results.

Weight training when combined with aerobic exercise, can boost your fitness and health level. You can do your weight training or weight lifting with or without use of a machine.

Benefits of Weight Lifting or Training

Apart from the overall health and fitness benefits, weight lifting benefits include:

a. Increased ligament strength

b. Increased muscles contractile strength

c. Increased muscle-fiber size

d. Increased tendon strength

e. A fit and healthier body that is less susceptible to injury

f. You look handsome and good

Ground Rules for Weight Training

To get the best out of your weight lifting exercise, observe the following rules:

a. Get your machines; equipment- such as dumb bells or bar bells, towels, etc; and benches ready

b. Always wipe the equipment, machines, and benches to use

c. Silence your handset, to avoid unnecessary distraction

d. Re-rack all the weight and dumb bells used

e. Must rest between 30 to 90 seconds for overall fitness

Weight Lifting Workout Guidelines

a. Carry out your workout for at least twice weekly

b. May perform 5 to 12 repetitions due to your goals, taking 4 to 5 seconds to complete a repetition in a slow manner

c. Rest 1 to 2 minutes between each exercise

d. Rest between 30 to 90 seconds between sets of each exercise or weight lifting

e. Use jump rope to warm up for 5 to 10 minutes

f. Stay hydrated. Drink enough water

Common Avoidable Mistakes

a. As you begin avoid using too much weight to avoid injury. Increase your weight gradually.

b. Avoid using underweight, when you know you can do more

c. Avoid lifting weights too fast

d. Avoid moving through repetitions too quickly and too fast

e. Avoid too much resting

f. Avoid not resting long enough

g. Failing to carry two towels. One for your post workout shower, one for sweat soaked equipment and bench

C. Adequate Rest and Physical Fitness

Proper Exercise Rest and Physical Fitness

There are certain ways to reaching your fitness goals through proper exercise rest.

Proper rest is an ingredient for physical fitness. Without proper rest, the body will breakdown in immunity and become illness or disease prone, thereby hindering total physical fitness.

Proper rest for physical fitness can be achieved by two ways, and these include exercise rest periods and sleep rest.

Proper Exercise Rest

When engaging in exercise, beware of over training or over doing a workout.

Over doing a workout takes place when your muscles have no required time to recover. Training too hard or too long is dangerous.

Desiring to rich your fitness goals or improve quickly enough at optimal levels, should not cause you to try to over train or get through in a day.

Over doing a workout leads to fatigue, injury, lowered performance, soreness, stiffness, and sudden heart attack. Train without allowing a recovery time, causes the muscles to become over stressed.

You must strike a balance between over doing a workout or training and workout effort. Allow breaks in your training to get needed recovery.

Don't workout too soon after a rigorous training session, so as to allow your muscles sufficient recovery time.

Over training results when you repeated undertake a cycle of bout or training, without allowing a complete recovery. Recovery from soreness of muscles can take up to three days rest.

When planning your fitness program, include rest periods, in order to give your muscles strength from recovery. Let your workout intensity, determine your recovery time.

With harder intensity of workout, more recovery time is needed to give you sufficient rest. Also, a less intensive workout requires a less rest period or recovery time.

You must avoid over doing a workout by stretching and warming up before training; watch your weight; have a two to three days breaks incorporated in your fitness or training plan; listen to your body talk to you; and slow down your training when you notice warning signs and symptoms of exercise or over training.

When recovery is needed, stop your exercise, drink water or other fluids, rest; take Glucose D or other carbohydrates to replenish lost glycogen in your body, especially liver and muscles, and sleep.

 If you must continue to do workout, engage in another exercise to avoid working the same muscles.

Proper Sleep Rest and Physical Fitness

Here are certain ways to reaching your fitness goals through proper sleep rest.

Proper rest is an ingredient for physical fitness. Without proper rest, the body will breakdown in immunity and become illness or disease prone, thereby hindering total physical fitness.

Proper rest for physical fitness can be achieved by two ways, and these include exercise rest periods and sleep rest.

As stated above, this section deals with proper sleep rest. Various steps to proper sleep rest are;

Get Set for Sleep Daily

On a daily basis, before you sleep, set the bed by removing everything including books and clothes, brush your teeth, set the alarm, and put on sleep dress.

Avoid Absence of Sleep Daily

Your body gets a lot of healing during sleep, especially during the time of a good night sleep or rest. Your body is prone to become weak or breakdown without a good night rest.

This breakdown begins from your body cells to organs and tissues. Absence of sleep rest causes restlessness, lack of concentration, weakness, irritable, etc.

Remove Remote causes of Sleeplessness

Many causes abound for not having a good night rest, such as body pains, environment, and illness. Still there must be adequate preparation for proper and adequate sleep or rest, so as to attain and maintain your goals for physical fitness.

Avoid or Stop all Activities

Your must sleep for about eight (8) hours daily, to give your body that needed rest for physical fitness.

In trying to sleep these numbers of hours, avoid stressful activities, exercise, browsing, computer operations, and TV viewing, reading, listening to radio, night or phone calls, working, homework or assignments. In about twenty to thirty minutes to sleep time, stop all activities.

Avoid Distractions

Get your room well prepared for sound sleep. Keep TV off your bedroom; make the environment conducive enough for sleep by switch off bright light and leaving dim lights to make the bedroom dark to avoid distraction, and providing proper temperature.

Eat and Drink Four Hours before Sleep

Also, don't eat and don't drink water in the last four hours before going to bed. Eating at this time before going to bed will cause your digestive system working or restless, while you are trying to get sleep rest.

Eat light foods, four hours before going to bed. Avoid drinking water after 6pm. Drinking water late will cause you to being awake often in order to ease yourself at the bathroom, thereby depriving you of sleep rest.

Avoid Taking Stimulants

Avoid caffeine, smoking, and alcohol before going to bed. Caffeine and smoking will keep you awake due to the stimulant called nicotine. Alcohol will make you sleep, but you will be awake frequently during the night.

Keep to a Regular Sleep Time

Try to keep to a regular bedtime and wake-up time. This will enable to have an adequate amount of sleep daily for the attainment of physical fitness.

Also avoid sleeping peels and other strong drugs. Take a hot bath and avoid worry and anxiety or manage your stress well.

With proper sleep rest as an ingredient for physical fitness, properly gotten, your fitness goals shall be achieved.

Living a Stress Free Life and Adequate Rest for Fitness

Stress symptoms include physical, social and mental indicators. Such symptoms include headache, sleeplessness and over-sleeping, extreme exhaustion and loss of appetite or over-appetite.

Stress can be managed to the extent of living a stress free life, all through the year. Stress is a state of high tension or pressure impacting hardship.

In Simple understanding, stress is anything that disturbs the natural balance between the body and the environment.

Stress management is the ability to maintain control when people, situations, circumstances and events, try to make excessive demands on an individual, almost to a breaking point.

The following top tips for living a stress free life would help you manage, control and prevent stress with ease:

1. Have A Good Health Education.

A good health education would enable you to have an insight into your various stress triggers and then devise a means of freedom or a means of coping with it.

2. Always live on the positive side of Life.

For you to cope with or manage stress, to the extend of being stress free, you must always think positive, speak positive, act positive and live positive. You must have nothing to do with worry and anxiety, in every form of situation.

3. Live A Healthy Live Daily.

To live a tress free life all through the year, you must think health and do the following:

i. Eat Balanced Diets.

Eat more of vegetables and fruits, up to 90% of your daily diet. They are full of minerals and vitamins, to help keep you energetic, strong and vibrant.

ii. Do Daily and Regular Exercise.

When you wake up from bed, stretch yourself, do jogging, go swimming, walk some distance, lift weights, do deep breathing daily, for about five minutes.

ii. Stop Or Avoid Harmful Habits.

Habits such as smoking of cigarette, drinking of alcohol and excess of caffeine are harmful to your health. Also, avoid self medication. These harmful habits often bring about stress. Get rid of them.

3. Be Free From Fear.

Do not be afraid what tomorrow may bring. Each morning, look up and move on through the day. In every situation, do not panic, just gain the control and you shall overcome.

4. Observe Good Attitudes Daily.

Your lifestyle must change in order to become stress free. As such, the following good attitudes should be observed:

i) Put a demand on relaxation daily

ii) Learn to communicate well

iii) Make contacts and friends

iv) Do something for others

v) Learn to smile and laugh too, to enable you release yourself, these when done would help you get your mind off yourself and your situations.

5. Get Enough Sleep.

Lack of sleep can bring about or worsen stress. You must sleep for eight (8) hours daily. Sleeping these hours enables your body to be refreshed and stress daily.

The services of a doctor or a professional counselor can be made use of, when you realize that stress is too hard on you.

D. Cleanliness and Physical Fitness

Personal Hygiene and Physical Fitness

In learning about physical fitness information about personal hygiene is important.

When your personal hygiene is right, you become looking good, clean, healthy, and happy.

The following steps would help you achieve the best in this respect.

1. Observe Regular and Daily Tooth Brushing.

Tooth brushing should start first thing in the morning. Brush your teeth two or three times daily, or after each meal.

Your tongue should be cleansed using your toothbrush. You must floss daily. There is the need also to see your dentist once a year.

2. Shower Twice Daily.

To look good and clean, you should shower daily, in the morning and at evening or night. If you involve in sports, sweat generating exercise, and in much dirty work, you need to shower at anytime you finish accomplishing such. Showering regularly helps keep away body odor.

Do not share your bathing towel. Use cotton swab to clean out excess wax in your ears.

Wash your face daily. Do so at least once a day, to remove all dirt that you may contact. This would also help keep wrinkles and pimples away.

Use a moisturizer to ensure that your face remains fresh and renewed.

3. Wash and Iron Your Clothes.

Wash your clothes after one or two times of wearing. Preferably when you sweat or notice your collar and some other parts become dirty. Ironing should also be carried out after washing and drying.

4. Keep Your Nails Trimmed.

Watch out and trim your nails when they grow. This would prevent debris or dirt underneath the nails.

5. Remove Unwanted Hair.

To look gook and clean, you need to get rid of unwanted hair on your face or other places you do not want them to appear.

Remove hair that grow out of your nostrils, ears, chin, upper and lower lips, etc. you can shave or use any other hair removal strategy, like hot waxing, laser hair removal, and electrolysis method, etc.

Have the hair on your head cut if grown. This is determined by the length of your hair. You can get your hair cut in every six to ten weeks.

Keep the hair on your head clean and conditioned, to enable it become strong and healthy. Do not wash it too frequently, to avoid making it dry and brittle.

6. Use Acne Prevention Cleanser.

If you have acne, use acne prevention cleanser to cover breakouts and prevent further acne. Do not squeeze or pick on the acne, this would worsen the situation.

Use oil blotting sheets for oily skin. Get the blotting sheets and soak out oil from your face throughout the day. This would enable your face look good and clean.

7. Take Care of Your Feet to Avoid Foot Troubles and Odor.

Air out your shoes after wearing and change socks regularly. Dust your shoes with baby powder. Do not wear shoes without socks, to avoid odor.

Dress cuts and burns if present. Cover all cuts, sores, and burns regularly. Better prevent yourself from having cuts and burns.

8. Avoid Strong Fragrance Or Perfumes.

Use soaps with less fragrance, which may cause offensive odor. Shower with less harsh or gentle soap.

Also, perfumes with strong fragrance, which produces strong and offensive odor, should be avoided. Maintain a clean personal hygiene, and there would be no need of perfumes.

9. Observe Regular Washing of Hands.

Most infections are got through the hands. So, wash your hands often to keep germs away.

Wash your hands with soap after touching saliva or vomit, after contact with animals, rubbish bins, the sick, after work, or after changing infants diaper, etc.

With the above tips for personal hygiene, you shall become good looking, clean, healthy, and fit.

E. Environment and Physical Fitness

Environmental pollution is dangerous to your health and fitness, because what happens outside would definitely affect what happens inside your body.

Harmful emissions from vehicles, generators, and other machines giving out fumes from their exhaust, go along way in affecting your environment.

Also, industrial and agricultural firms dump their wastes which are contaminants to our environment. Some of these contaminants are deposited in our open waters.

Smoke from exhaust and smokers are harmful to the body when inhaled, because it is made up of a harmful gas called carbon monoxide.

Automobile emissions add up to the build up of carbon dioxide. This becomes a problem when the volume becomes more than what is needed.

Your health can be affected greatly by the accumulation of these pollutants, leading to cancer and other infectious diseases.

In some places, human waste which is used for fertilizer contains toxins. When these toxins are absorbed by plants and we eat the plants, health problems may arise.

Water can be contaminated with medicines from many patients, like hepatitis patients. In addition, toxic waste from feces goes along way to affect one's health, if such water is consumed.

Pesticides and fertilizer residues from both are water and food, becomes dangerous when taken in. In some cosmetics and medicines, toxins additives and other substances are dangerous to your health.

Many are unaware of the harmful effects of caffeine that is being consumed daily by many. Also, Cigarette and marijuana are dangerous producers of harmful smoke that may affect the body.

Sulfur and nitrogen oxides from coal burning equipment and factories, get combined in the atmosphere and drop as rain, snow, and dust. This leads to environmental destruction which may affect your health.

The use of pesticides and chemical fertilizers made up of nitrogen, phosphorus, and potassium, produces nitrates from runoffs or irrigation, which end up in rivers, ponds, and wells, leading to water contamination. This makes the water unfit for human and animal consumption.

Most processed foods have a higher concentration of pesticides. This is harmful to your health and fitness. Also, food coloring and preservatives that are used for most processed foods are dangerous to your health.

Environmental pollution has penetrated indoors, sending in toxins, such as benzene, formaldehyde, and chloroform.

In trying to keep the home in an air tight condition, pollution arises. This is just sealing of us with pollutants which are dangerous to health.

Formaldehyde is known to cause headache, eye irritation, depression, and asthma.

We cannot live without air. We need oxygen for our survival. The oxygen we take in enters our blood system, and is being transported to various cells of the body, to generate energy for our livelihood.

As such we need to take care of the air we breathe and our general environment. This would go along way to keeps our body healthy and free from the various harmful effects of environmental pollution.

You have to watch your environment, and make sure that the various toxins, and pollutants, that many have been caught up with, do not have an entrance into your body. By this you would be free and maintain a good fitness level.

F. Medication and Physical Fitness

Most individuals suffer from chronic illness that can be prevented through regular physical activity, exercise, and fitness.

There are many diseases that can be prevented and even cured without medication. As we have already mentioned that common cold can be prevented and even cure through regular exercise habit.

Physical activity also aids the prevention of heart disease by improving one's cholesterol level. Other preventable diseases through physical activity are high blood pressure, non-insulin dependent diabetes mellitus, osteoarthritis, osteoporosis, obesity, weakened immune system, rheumatoid arthritis, etc.

The truth is that those in the medical profession know this, but will never promote it, because nobody will patronize them. People want to hear them say 'buy and take this drug and your common cold will go in the next hour'.

Experts have proven that physical activity is known to enhance longevity and the quality of life of people of all ages. Also, that those who engage in physical activity have less accidents and die less.

Smoking and alcohol consumption can harm your fitness level and health. Self medication and wrong use of drugs can also harm your physical fitness.

You can reach and achieve a lifetime of physical fitness when you learn and practice the above measures. You would become good looking, healthy, and physically fit.

To your physical fitness

www.ingramcontent.com/pod-product-compliance
Lightning Source LLC
Chambersburg PA
CBHW071213280526
45787CB00002B/670